EMPOWERING HEALTH

Managing High Blood Pressure Made Simple

DR. MATAMI JAMES

CONTENTS

4

INTRODUCTION

High blood pressure, also known as hypertension, is a condition in which the force of blood pushing against the walls of your arteries is consistently too high. This condition can be very dangerous, as it can damage your blood vessels and lead to serious health problems such as heart disease, stroke, and kidney failure.

It is important to understand high blood pressure because it is one of the most common health conditions in the world, affecting millions of people of all ages and backgrounds. In fact, according to the World Health Organization, high blood pressure is responsible for more deaths worldwide than any other single risk factor.

The purpose of this book is to provide you with a comprehensive understanding of high blood pressure, its causes, effects, diagnosis, treatment, prevention, and management. By reading this book, you will be able to:

- Recognize the signs and symptoms of high blood pressure

- Understand the causes and risk factors for high blood pressure

- Learn how high blood pressure affects the body and can lead to other health problems

- Identify the different types of high blood pressure

- Know how high blood pressure is diagnosed and treated

- Understand the importance of prevention and management strategies

- Gain insights into living with high blood pressure and coping with its emotional and psychological effects

This book is structured in a way that will allow you to easily navigate the information presented and find what you need to know. Each chapter builds on the previous one, providing you with a complete understanding of high blood pressure and how to manage it.

UNDERSTANDING HIGH BLOOD PRESSURE

In this chapter, we will explore the definition of high blood pressure, how it is measured, and the various causes and risk factors associated with this condition. We will also discuss the different types of high blood pressure.

Definition and Measurement of High Blood Pressure

Blood pressure is measured in millimeters of mercury (mmHg) and consists of two numbers: systolic pressure and diastolic pressure. Systolic pressure is the force of blood against the arterial walls when the heart beats, while diastolic pressure is the force of blood when the heart is at rest between beats.

High blood pressure is generally defined as a systolic pressure reading of 140 mmHg or higher, and/or a diastolic pressure reading of 90 mmHg or higher. However, high blood pressure can also be diagnosed if your blood pressure is consistently elevated over time, even if it is not in the hypertensive range.

Causes and Risk Factors for High Blood Pressure
There are many factors that can contribute to the development of high blood pressure, including:

- Genetics: Family history of high blood pressure can increase your risk.

- Age: Blood vessels become less flexible and more prone to narrowing as you age, which can increase your risk.

- Lifestyle factors: Unhealthy diet, lack of physical activity, and being overweight or obese can increase your risk.

- Smoking: Nicotine in cigarettes can raise your blood pressure and damage your blood vessels.

- Stress: Chronic stress can cause your body to release hormones that increase your blood pressure.

- Certain medical conditions: Diabetes, kidney disease, and sleep apnea can increase your risk of developing high blood pressure.

Types of High Blood Pressure

There are two main types of high blood pressure: primary hypertension and secondary hypertension.

Primary hypertension, also known as essential hypertension, is the most common type of high blood pressure and has no identifiable cause. Secondary hypertension, on the other hand, is caused by an underlying medical condition or medication.

EFFECTS OF HIGH BLOOD PRESSURE

High blood pressure is a serious health condition that can have harmful effects on the body. In this chapter, we will discuss the various ways that high blood pressure can affect your health and how it can lead to other health problems.

Effects of High Blood Pressure

High blood pressure can cause damage to your blood vessels, which can lead to:

Atherosclerosis: A buildup of plaque in the arteries that can narrow or block blood flow, leading to heart attack or stroke.

Arterial aneurysm: A bulge in the wall of an artery that can rupture and cause internal bleeding.

Kidney damage: High blood pressure can damage the kidneys and lead to kidney failure.

Vision loss: High blood pressure can damage the blood vessels in the eyes and lead to vision loss.

Sexual dysfunction: High blood pressure can reduce blood flow to the genital area, leading to erectile dysfunction in men and decreased libido in women.

High Blood Pressure and Other Health Problems
High blood pressure can also increase your risk of developing other health problems, including:

Heart disease: High blood pressure is a major risk factor for heart disease, including heart attack, heart failure, and arrhythmias.

Stroke: High blood pressure can increase your risk of stroke by damaging blood vessels in the brain.

Diabetes: High blood pressure can increase your risk of developing type 2 diabetes.

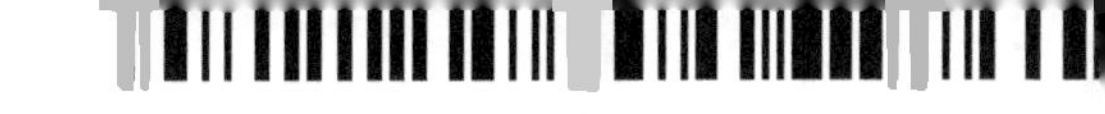

Metabolic syndrome: High blood pressure is one of the five components of metabolic syndrome, a group of conditions that increase your risk of heart disease, stroke, and diabetes.

Cognitive decline: High blood pressure can increase your risk of cognitive decline and dementia.

DIAGNOSIS AND TREATMENT

In this chapter, we will discuss how high blood pressure is diagnosed and the various treatment options available. We will also explore the potential side effects of medications used to treat high blood pressure.

Diagnosis of High Blood Pressure

High blood pressure is typically diagnosed through a blood pressure measurement taken by a healthcare professional. This can be done at a doctor's office, clinic, or pharmacy. To diagnose high blood pressure, a healthcare professional will take two or more readings on separate occasions and average the results.

In some cases, a healthcare professional may recommend additional tests to determine the cause of high blood pressure or to check for related health problems.

There are various treatment options available for high blood pressure, including lifestyle changes and medications.

Lifestyle changes can include:

- Eating a healthy diet low in sodium and rich in fruits, vegetables, and whole grains

- Maintaining a healthy weight

- Regular exercise

- Limiting alcohol consumption

- Quitting smoking

In some cases, medication may be necessary to lower high blood pressure. There are several types of medications used to treat high blood pressure, including:

- Diuretics: These medications help the body get rid of excess water and salt, which can lower blood pressure.

- Beta-blockers: These medications reduce the workload on the heart by slowing the heart rate and reducing the force of contractions.

- ACE inhibitors: These medications help relax blood vessels by preventing the production of a hormone that narrows blood vessels.

- Calcium channel blockers: These medications help relax blood vessels by preventing calcium from entering the cells of the heart and blood vessels.

Potential Side Effects of Medications

While medications can be effective in treating high blood pressure, they can also have potential side effects. Some common side effects of blood pressure medications include:

- Dizziness

- Fatigue

- Headaches

- Nausea

- Erectile dysfunction

- Dry cough

It is important to talk to your healthcare professional about the potential side effects of any medication you are prescribed.

PREVENTION AND MANAGEMENT

In this chapter, we will discuss the steps that can be taken to prevent high blood pressure and the lifestyle changes that can be made to manage high blood pressure. We will also explore the importance of monitoring blood pressure regularly.

Prevention of High Blood Pressure

While there are risk factors for high blood pressure that cannot be controlled, such as age, family history, and genetics, there are steps that can be taken to prevent high blood pressure. These steps include:

Maintaining a healthy weight

Eating a healthy diet low in sodium and rich in fruits, vegetables, and whole grains

- Regular exercise

- Limiting alcohol consumption

- Quitting smoking

- Managing stress

Management of High Blood Pressure

For those with high blood pressure, lifestyle changes can be an effective way to manage blood pressure. Some lifestyle changes that can help manage high blood pressure include:

- Eating a healthy diet low in sodium and rich in fruits, vegetables, and whole grains

- Regular exercise

- Limiting alcohol consumption

- Quitting smoking

- Managing stress

- Taking prescribed medications as directed by a healthcare professional

It is important to work with a healthcare professional to develop a personalized plan to manage high blood pressure.

Monitoring Blood Pressure

Regular monitoring of blood pressure is important for the prevention and management of high blood pressure. Blood pressure should be checked at least once a year for those with normal blood pressure levels and more frequently for those with high blood pressure.

Monitoring blood pressure can be done at home using a home blood pressure monitor or at a healthcare professional's office. It is important to follow the instructions for taking blood pressure measurements and to record the results.

LIVING WITH HIGH BLOOD PRESSURE

In this chapter, we will discuss strategies for coping with the emotional and psychological effects of high blood pressure, tips for managing daily life with high blood pressure, and the importance of support from family and friends.

Coping with the Emotional and Psychological Effects of High Blood Pressure

High blood pressure can have a significant impact on a person's emotional and psychological well-being. It can be stressful to manage a chronic condition and to constantly monitor blood pressure. Some strategies for coping with the emotional and psychological effects of high blood pressure include:

- Seeking support from family and friends

- Joining a support group

- Practicing stress-reducing techniques such as meditation, yoga, or deep breathing exercises

- Speaking with a mental health professional

Managing Daily Life with High Blood Pressure

Managing daily life with high blood pressure requires making healthy choices and developing a routine that works for you. Some tips for managing daily life with high blood pressure include:

- Eating a healthy diet low in sodium and rich in fruits, vegetables, and whole grains

- Regular exercise

- Taking medications as prescribed by a healthcare professional

- Monitoring blood pressure regularly

- Quitting smoking and limiting alcohol consumption

- Managing stress

The support of family and friends can be helpful for those living with high blood pressure. Family and friends can offer emotional support, encouragement, and assistance in making healthy choices. It is important to educate family and friends about high blood pressure and how they can be supportive.

CONCLUSION

In this final chapter, we will provide a recap of the key points discussed in the book and offer some final thoughts and advice for readers living with high blood pressure.

Recap of Key Points

In this book, we have discussed what high blood pressure is and why it is important to understand it. We have explored the causes, risk factors, and types of high blood pressure, as well as its harmful effects on the body and its potential to lead to other health problems. We have also discussed how high blood pressure is diagnosed and treated, as well as the lifestyle changes and medications that can be used to manage it.

Additionally, we have provided tips for preventing and managing high blood pressure, including the importance of monitoring blood pressure regularly.

Finally, we have discussed strategies for coping with the emotional and psychological effects of high blood pressure, as well as the importance of support from family and friends.

If you are living with high blood pressure, it is important to remember that you are not alone. Millions of people around the world are managing this condition, and with proper management, you can lead a healthy and fulfilling life.

It is essential to work closely with your healthcare team to manage your high blood pressure. This includes following a healthy diet, getting regular exercise, taking medications as prescribed, and monitoring your blood pressure regularly.

Additionally, it is important to make lifestyle changes that can help prevent or manage high blood pressure.

These changes may include reducing your sodium intake, quitting smoking, and limiting your alcohol consumption.

Finally, we encourage you to seek support from family, friends, or a support group. Managing high blood pressure can be challenging, but with the right resources and support, it is possible to live a healthy and fulfilling life.

In closing, we hope that this book has provided you with valuable information about high blood pressure and its management. By working closely with your healthcare team and making healthy choices, you can take control of your health and lead a happy, healthy life.